THE SECRET TO BEAUTIFUL NATURAL NAILS

How to Say Goodbye to Peeling Nails, and Artificial Nails Forever!

Alicia Lyons

Illustrations by Dawn Loberg

Illustrations by Dawn Loberg
Photo credit: Deb Weinkauff/Sedona Monthly

This book was printed in the United States of America.

To order additional copies of this book, contact:
Xlibris Corporation
1-888-795-4274
www.Xlibris.com
Orders@Xlibris.com
49911

Contents

DEDICATION

This book is dedicated to Bob. Without his understanding, support and love throughout all these years, this information would not be possible.

This book is also dedicated to all the clients (friends) that I have worked with throughout the years. Thank you for all your patience and kindness and for helping me grow to become the professional that I am today.

"Everything should be as simple as possible, but no simpler."
-**Albert Einstein**

"The only interesting answers are those which destroy the questions."
-**Susan Sontag b. 1933**
American writer and social critic

"Year by year, the complexities of this world grow more bewildering, and so each year we need all the more to see peace and comfort in joyful simplicities."
-**Women's Home Companion**
December 1935

PREFACE

Why Educate the Public

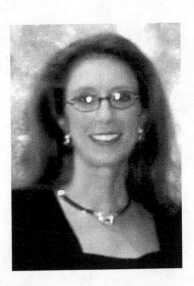

Hi, my name is Alicia Lyons. I've been a manicurist since 1982. I'm what people in my profession call a veteran nail tech. However, back then, we were called ourselves manicurists and not nail techs. Of course, this is when the ladies of leisure would come into the salon and have a basic manicure while they were sitting under the dryer with their hair in curlers.

I've seen the nail industry change in dramatic ways. I even had clients that wanted me to go to the dental supply store to get product to put on their nails, this would be the MMA acrylics that are so unhealthy. I've seen former dental supply companies become nail supply companies. Do the names Creative Nail Design and OPI ring a bell? I've seen the birth of the "French Manicure". I could never figure out what was wrong with the white pencil we used to use under the nail, it was more natural looking then painting white on the top of the nail.

I've also seen the birth of "discount nail salons", the places that do your nails so quick and cheaply that, in some cases, the nail tech doesn't take time to sanitize things properly. In the beginning, they were not as numerous as they are now. Now, they are everywhere. The discount nail salon has its place in today's society because they are fast and cheap, but dirty nail techs that injure their clients do not.

Unsanitary nail techs have become the number one health concern of the beauty industry. And don't be too surprised to find these unclean technicians in upscale salons and spas. Many states have problems keeping up with the complaints that the consumers have, let alone some of the difficulties surrounding epidemics, due to some of their sanitation procedures. It's time that they cleaned up their act! Let's tell them it is not okay to rip off our nails and then wonder why we cry out in pain. It is because of all the complaints that I have heard through the years from clients who have gone to these technicians and had bad experiences . . . It is because there are not enough state inspectors out there to deal quickly with the problems that keep occurring . . . It is because some clients don't even know if their technician is performing the service in a legal or clean manner . . . It is because of my long history of doing nails and knowing what is the right way to perform a service, sanitize my implements, and treat a client with care and respect, that I've decided that it is time to make uncaring, dirty nail techs clean up their act. Now, I won't say that all nail technicians are bad (heck, I've been one for 25 years) there are a lot of very good ones out there, and some of them work in discount nail salons. The trick is to find the good nail techs. So if you're tired of wondering how clean your nail technician is, or if your tired of constantly saying "Ouch, you're hurting me!" I have got the perfect answer for you. This publication is going to help you say goodbye to artificial nails, goodbye to that dirty nail tech, and hello to beautiful, healthy, natural nails. This publication will help you to achieve this on your own. You don't need to go to a dirty nail tech anymore.

Please note, this publication is for the beautification of the nails and is not meant to treat any diseases or maladies. If you have any concerns of this nature, I highly recommend that you see a physician.

Introduction to Natural Nail Care

Throughout the years of being in this profession, people have always asked me, "What is the best way to grow my nails long and healthy? "Well," I reply, "the best way to grow your nails long and healthy is . . ." Of course, at this time, all heads turn, ears leaning in to gain some unknown knowledge from a seasoned nail professional. "First, you need to go to a bedding or house wares store. It doesn't matter if you go to Bed, Bath & Beyond or if you go to Wal-Mart," (here is where I add a pregnant pause just because I can't help myself) "any place you feel you can find a big square satin or silk pillow. It needs to be satin or silk, preferably silk." (another loaded pause) "It doesn't matter what color you choose, if you can find your favorite color, go with that, to heck with your current home decor. After you get this pillow, you need to take it home and place it in the middle of the floor, away from as many things as possible. Next, I want you to sit on this pillow and don't touch a damn thing, NOTHING! That is the way to grow your nails long and healthy."

But seriously, most women are not ladies of leisure. Most of us do a lot of typing, housework with nasty chemicals, gardening and many more things that harm our nails and wear them down. Yes, I said, wear down. Keep in mind that everything you touch acts as a natural nail file. Have you ever wondered why your ring finger and pinkie fingers grow faster than your other fingers? They don't! In fact, your middle finger grows the fastest but it is always getting bumped and broken down, especially when you hit it while you're cleaning your kitchen counter or snap it off on the car door. To be honest, most fingernails grow about a quarter of an inch a month. This is an average based on your metabolism. In fact, I'm certain most of you never realized they could grow that fast. The big trick is; "How do I get my nails to not wear away as fast?" Well I'm going to tell you all the little secrets that some nail techs don't know or can't explain. How do you get your nails to be strong, long, healthy and beautiful? The true secret is, it's not a quick fix and it takes a little effort on your part. The first and probably the hardest rule to adhere to is;

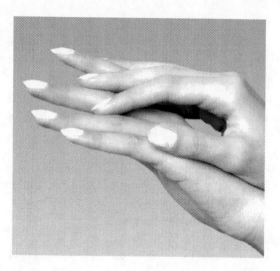

"Your nails are jewels *not* tools.

Treat them as such"

I heard an old boss say this to me and I had to agree. Even most men will say, "Use the right tool for the job." I hate to say this, ladies, but your nail on your forefinger doesn't look like a screwdriver. We've *all* done this or something like it, now we need to stop it.

A beautiful, healthy nail, needs to be STRONG *and* FLEXIBLE. Also, for a beautifully manicured hand, all your nails should be about the same length. I know a lot of women, especially younger women and teens who will usually have a few nails really long, mostly the ring and pinkie fingers. They just can't seem to part with them. "It took me so long to grow and I really don't want to cut it down." is what I usually have heard from most of these girls. I'm sorry to say, this is not considered "well manicured". It just looks uneven. But if you follow a few simple rules, you can have beautiful, well manicured hands, and all your nails can be longer and healthier.

The answer to beautiful natural nails comes with understanding how to shape, oil and polish your nails. In order to do this, you must first understand that the nails you possess are the nails you were born with. The structure of the nails you have and how they can be improved upon is fundamental in what we will be deal with here in this book. Now, how do you do it? First, have you worn artificial nails lately? Have your nails been natural for at least six months or more? We will explain a little about artificial nails then we will determine the current condition of your nails.

Artificial Nails

Dangers of Artificial Nails

As most people know, artificial nails can look very lovely but only when they are very uniform in appearance and not thick or lumpy. But there are also hidden problems when wearing artificial nails. What a lot of people don't know is that it doesn't matter if you have acrylic, gel nails or even silk wraps, they all cause damage to the natural nail.

Another problem is that it is very easy, as most people know, to get a bacterial infection on or under the nail. Most people know these to be "Greenies" or "Fungus Infection". First let me explain what these are. They are both bacterial infections.

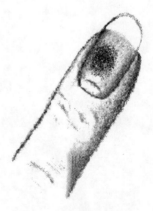

- "Greenie"—bacteria get in between the natural fingernail and the artificial nail. The green is a byproduct of the bacteria eating the natural oils between the two. The longer the bacterium sits between the natural nail and the artificial nail, the darker it becomes. The green will stain the natural nail and the only way to remove the green (after removing the artificial nail) is to buff it off. This may not be a good idea if the nail is deeply stained because the natural nail is only so thick and the staining may go through to the nail bed. Buffing deeply will only injure the nail further.

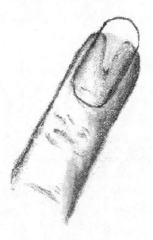

- "Fungus Infection"—is a misnomer; on the fingernails, it is really a bacterial infection. When a nail becomes injured, whether by a nail drill, improper filing, improper nail cleaning, nail picking, or any other numerous ways, the infection gets into the bed of the nail and separates the nail bed from the fingernail itself.

The only way to get rid of these infections is to let them grow out. The "Greenie" needs to have the artificial nail removed and gently buffed. The "Fungus Infection" needs an antibacterial treatment like Tea Tree Oil, White Iodine or any of the numerous "antifungal" nail treatments that you find over the counter. There are numerous different products and companies out there with very effective treatments. However, I have noticed that most clients use these products on an inconsistent basis. They will treat their nail only once a day and then stop treatment when it looks like the infection is growing out. This is not the way to get rid of the infection. You must treat the infected nail several times per day as directed by the manufacturer, usually 2-3 times per day, and continue to do so until the infection is totally grown out. This information cannot be stressed enough.

You cannot easily get a real fungus infection on your fingernail because it would need to stay damp and in the dark, the way your feet are when they are in socks. Most infections that happen on the fingernails due to artificial nails are bacterial in character.

Another problem some people have with artificial nails is allergic reactions. With allergic reactions, most people develop itching, redness and swelling around the cuticle area. Severe cases will include the nail separating from the nail bed. Allergic reactions will only get worse the more you wear artificial nails. If you take the acrylic or gel off your nail and then try to put nails back on, albeit it has been a year or ten years, your allergic reaction will be the same or worse. These reactions usually happen with acrylic and gel nails and not as much with glue or resin based products.

There is an acrylic liquid that increases the chance of allergic reaction called MMA, or Methyl Methacrylate. Some people call it "dental acrylics" or "porcelain nails". The FDA had received so many complaints that they asked manufactures to change the formulations. Most manufacturers reformulated their products to the less dangerous EMA, Ethel Methacrylate, which is less harmful. Most, if not all, states have made it illegal to use MMA in a nail salon. However, there are still some dubious nail techs that continue to use MMA. How can you tell if you have MMA Acrylics versus EMA Acrylics? Here are some signs to be aware of:

- MMA Acrylic nails will not soak off easily
- MMA Acrylics are extremely hard and difficult to file
- MMA liquid has a stronger odor than EMA liquid

Advantages of Artificial Nails

There are advantages for some people to wear artificial nails, but this is only when all other options have been visited. Some of the reasons are:

- They bite their nails and get artificial nails to prevent them from biting. It helps them to have something that automatically looks attractive in order to prevent them from biting their nails. Yet some of these people will still bite the artificial nails off.
- To minimize abnormalities such as:

  - Nails that are not straight—artificial nails can make crooked nails look straighter

- Nails that have very deep ridges that split down the center into the skin—artificial nails make them look smooth and hold the nail together
- Ski-Jump nails look flatter or even have a natural curve downward with artificial nails

- People who are "Bulls in a China Shop" will get artificial nails. They continually break their natural nails because they are exceedingly hard on their natural nails.

Lifting

Your overall health and what you do with your hands will be reflected in your nails. If you are hard on your hands, you will usually have lifting on the nails that you use most often. If you notice regular lifting on a specific nail, it is usually because you are using that nail in a way that causes it to lift. Closely observe what you do with that nail or nails in between your fill-ins. For instance, a client of mine kept loosing her middle nail on her right hand. After numerous attempts to make the nail adhere, I asked my client to watch what she may be doing with that nail that might make it lift. What we learned was that she was using that finger very roughly on her adding machine and she used the adding machine on a very regular basis. This was obviously the cause of the lifting. Also, going too long between your fills can increase your chance of lifting.

If your health is suffering, all your artificial nails will lift more than usual. Some conditions, like thyroid conditions and people on chemotherapy, will have extreme cases of lifting. This is not due to the technician but is because your nail is in such an unhealthy state that the artificial nail cannot adhere properly. If you have lifting with your artificial nails and your technician has truly tried everything to try to adhere the product, then I suggest that you see a physician. There might be a symptomatic cause for the lifting that only your physician can help diagnose. Keep in mind that some conditions could be as simple as a vitamin or mineral deficiency, but it is always a good idea to have a doctor look at any changes that may not seem normal.

Types of Artificial Nails

Most people think that all artificial nails are similar in how they react to the nails. There are also some misnomers about the different types of artificial nails. One of the most common is that one type of artificial nail is less damaging than another. This is not always true. In most cases, the damage to the natural nail occurs when the nail is put on, if it lifts and when it is filled. What causes the damage is how many layers of nail plate are damaged. When the artificial nail is first put on, how much of the natural nail is roughed up or "buffed" to make sure the product adheres to the nail. If the nail lifts easily, this is a problem. Every time your nail lifts, it damages the natural nail by damaging the nail plate yet again. When you fill your nail, any lifted product needs to be removed (this is optimal to prevent the nail from having "fill lines"), then the new nail that has grown out needs to be roughed up or "buffed" again to be certain that the new product adheres to the natural nail.

What are the differences between the different types of artificial nails? Here is a list of the differences.

Acrylic

This is when a liquid and a powder are mixed together and placed on the nail. Acrylic nails will soak off in Artificial Nail Remover or Acetone. The dust particles also seem larger when filed. An EMA type of acrylic nail will soak off in less time than an MMA acrylic nail.

Gel

Gel nails are applied exactly as it sounds, it is a gel type substance applied to the nail, then it is "cured" in a UV (Ultra Violet) light. Don't be fooled by technicians that say that you have Gel Nails when you have Acrylic Nails with a Gel Sealer. A Gel sealer is a product that is applied at the end of a service that fills in scratches and fine lines and leaves a high gloss. Another way to determine if you have gels is; Gel Nails normally *DO NOT* soak off. They can only be filed off. The dust particles for Gel nails are also much smaller and easier to file than acrylic. Be aware that many discount salons tell you that their putting on Gel Nails, but in reality they give you Acrylic nails with a Gel Sealer. File off the Sealer and your nails will soak off in Artificial Nail Remover or Acetone.

Silk/Fiberglass Wrap

Silk wraps have a very fine mesh, while Fiberglass wraps have a wider mesh. Both are applied with a glue or resin based product. Resin/Glue products do not have the adhesion properties that acrylic or gel do. However, in reality, there is no need to rough up the nail too much if the nail won't adhere as well in the first place.

Glue/Resin Product

Glue/Resin products are usually used with Silk/Fiberglass Wraps. Sometimes these products work well when used with an Acrylic filler powder. The Glue/Resin is applied then the filler powder is dusted over the wet Glue/Resin. This adds bulk to the nail and is beneficial when it is done over a crack in the nail.

No Pain Approach to Removing Artificial Nails

Removing artificial nails differs depending on the type of artificial nail that you have. Remember that extreme care is needed to remove artificial nails to minimize the damage. If you pick or rip the nails off, you will damage the nail and potentially injure your finger(s). You will need to pay close attention while filing to be certain that you are filing off the artificial nail and not the natural nail. If you file the natural nail too much, you will thin and weaken it. This will only increase the damage and the time of keeping them shorter because they will not be able to handle the stress of every day use.

To remove artificial nails, you will need the following:

- several files; a medium and a fine file
- a buffer as you get closer to the natural nail.
- Orangewood stick to remove the bulk of the product being soaked off
- Cotton
- Foil

Saturate some cotton, enough to cover the nail being removed, with some Acetone or Artificial Nail Remover. Place your finger on foil that is cut large enough to fit around the tip of your finger, and then place the saturated cotton on the nail to be removed. Wrap the foil around the finger (shiny side in) so that the liquid on the cotton stays inside the foil. When you wrap the foil around the finger with the shiny side in, it helps to keep your body heat in and keep the acetone warm. This technique helps in the faster removal of the nail. Artificial nail removal works best if you scrape off the excess product 2-3 times in between the beginning time and the ending time.

Use the following chart to determine if you need product remover and the approximate times needed to remove the artificial nail. If the time to soak off your nails is longer for the acrylic than stated, you may have MMA acrylic.

Type of Nail	Thickness	Use of Acetone or Artificial Nail Remover	Approximate Removal Time
Gel	Thick	No - File only	45 min - 1 hr
Gel	Medium	No - File only	30 - 45 min
Gel	Thin	No - File only	20 - 40 min
Acrylic	Extra Thick	Yes	1 - 1 ½ hr
Acrylic	Thick	Yes	45 min - 1 hr
Acrylic	Medium	Yes	30 - 45 min
Acrylic	Thin	Yes	20 - 40 min
Silk/Fiberglass Wrap	Thick	Yes	30 - 45 min
Silk/Fiberglass Wrap	Medium	Yes	20 - 40 min
Silk/Fiberglass Wrap	Thin	Yes	10 - 15 min
Glue/Resin w/Acrylic Powder	Full Nail - Thick	Yes	1 - 1 1/2 hr
Glue/Resin w/Acrylic Powder	Full Nail - Medium	Yes	45 min - 1 hr
Glue/Resin w/Acrylic Powder	Full Nail - Thin	Yes	30 - 45 min
Glue/Resin w/Acrylic Powder	Nail Repair	Yes	5 - 10 min

Artificial Nail Recovery

After you remove your artificial nails, you'll need to be patient and learn to create good nail care habits. It is going to take four to six months, for some people up to eight months, for your nails to completely grow out. But if you follow the directions in this book, keeping oil on your nails, keeping them filed short until they can withstand a little more length and keep polish on at all times, you can have better nails than what you started with before your artificial nails were put on. But in order to do this, you'll need to first understand a few things about the natural nail.

Nail Structure & Strength

You need to recognize that the nails, both their shape and thickness, that you have (excluding artificial nail damage) are a genetic trait. There is nothing that you can do to change this simple fact. You need to understand what your genetics tell you about your nails and how to assist them to be more of what you want them to be. And you need to be *reasonable* with this. There are also a few things you need to understand about the nail structure so you will understand the concepts I'll be explaining.

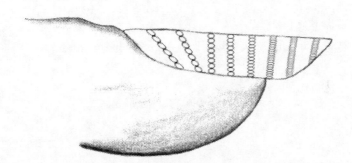

Consider your nails are literally layers of flattened cells stacked one on top of another. This is what we call a nail plate. An average nail has hundreds of cells stacked one on top of the other. The fatter the cells, the more moisture there is in them, the flatter they are, the dryer they are. The fatter cells have more moisture and are the youngest cells. These cells start to form a nail at an area called the matrix, which is nearest to your cuticle. The "Nail Moon" is where the nail cells are plump with moisture. As the nail cells grow out, they loose moisture and flatten out. All of these cells are held together with a cement like protein called keratin. It is when this cement is broken down at the tip of the nail that we get peeling. We will be addressing the issue of how to we prevent this protein from being broken down later.

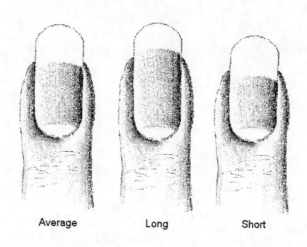

Average   Long   Short

Genetically, some people have long nail beds and some people have short nail beds. For those not familiar with "nail jargon", the nail bed is the pink part of your nail that is attached to your skin. If you have long nail beds, consider yourself very lucky. Even if your nails are filed short on the free edge (the white part of the nail) they will still look long when painted.

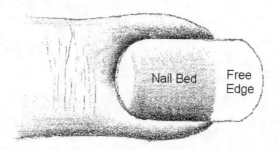

I should also point out that there are different shape nails besides the length of the nail bed that play an important part in how durable your nails are. This is because the nail has a stress area. The stress area is where the skin leaves the sides of the nail and where the nail will probably break if hit. Understanding your own genetic makeup allows you to determine how vulnerable your nails are to breaking. This will also help you to understand how long you can wear your nail before it is liable to break.

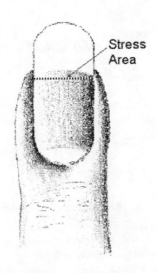

If you are looking at the side view of the nail, you may notice a slight downward slope to your nail; this is preferred for a good stress area. The nails tend to be more vulnerable to breaking when they are flatter.

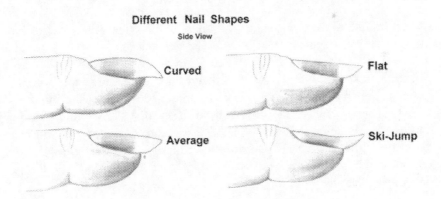

C-Curve

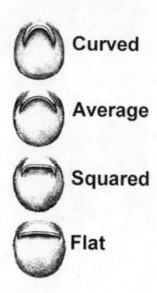

Curved

Average

Squared

Flat

Next, look down the barrel of the finger to determine your C-curve. If your C-curve is "Curved" as shown on the chart, then you have a better stress area than most. Again, flatter nails tend to be more vulnerable to breaking. There are also nails that bend sharply down on one side. This is usually, genetic or because of damage to the matrix of the nail. This is a condition which cannot be changed.

Of course there is also nail thickness. This is definitely beneficial. However, if you are just getting over acrylic, gel nails or even silk wraps then your nails are thin from damage. There is no sure fire way to get your nails thicker. Thicker nails only happen with age and, on the fingers, it is usually not extremely obvious. The best way I can describe it is as a callusing of the nail. This is why toenails get thick, they rub on the tips/tops of your shoes day in, and day out, year after year. I'm also sure that many of you have heard the old wives tale. If you drink gelatin your nails will grow thicker. Unfortunately, this is only true if you drink 8 packets of Knox ® Gelatin per day for the rest of your life.

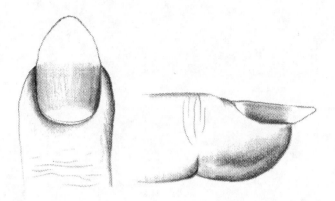

Short & Flat

For those of you who have thin nails on a short nail bed, with a flat C-curve and ski jump nails, I'm afraid that you have a challenge to create length on your nail. It is usually best to keep your nails a little shorter and try the different shapes for your nails. The best shape for your type of nail is usually a short (but not too short) oval. Don't despair; there is still hope for beautiful manicured hands.

Now that you have established your nails for their genetic characteristics, lets move on to what your lifestyle dictates.

Health & Other Factors

Your overall health will be reflected in your nails. It is always a good idea to take supplements when you are trying to grow healthy nails. Your age also plays a big part in how strong and how flexible your nails are. The younger you are, generally, your nails are thinner and tear easy, but they are more flexible. The older you are, your nails are usually dryer, thicker and sometimes less flexible. White patches on the surface of the nail and peeling nails are usually the result of overly dry nails. There can also be vertical or horizontal ridges.

Brittle nails, the white patches on the surface of the nail, severe peeling of the nails, occur with age. There have been studies done that show taking biotin supplements daily help improve this condition. Daily doses of 2.5 mg of biotin reduce brittle nails and helps increase nail thickness. Results will not show for approximately 6 months, the time that it takes for the nail to grow out from the nail matrix to the free edge.

Vertical ridges usually happen when the nails dry out, in other words, there is not a lot of oil in your nail holding in the nail's moisture content. They can also occur when there has been trauma to the matrix (area from where the nail grows). Very deep ridges can be caused by warts or tumors. We will help you to understand how to minimize minor ridges with cuticle oil.

Nail Ridges

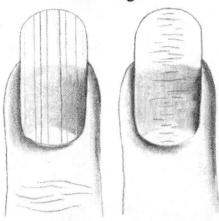

Vertical   **Horizontal**

Horizontal ridges usually happen when there has been damage to the nail matrix due to infection or physical damage. If the person has a nervous habit such as "worrying" (rubbing incessantly) at their fingers, they will usually find ridges on the fingers that they play with, usually this will be on the thumb/forefinger. These types of ridges can go away if the person stops the nervous habit. Picking at the cuticle area of a nail will also cause horizontal ridging if the person gets an infection in the cuticle. If the person has had an infection, the ridges will not go away. If you have horizontal ridges on *all* of your nails, please see a physician as this can be symptomatic of something more complex. Conditions such as, psoriasis or eczema can cause small horizontal pits in the nails. It is always best to see a physician if you notice ridging or pitting on all your nails.

Also, if you have been on a strict diet and your nutrition has suffered in any way it will show in your nails. Sometimes the effects of an internal health issue will usually not be noticed for about six months after the condition starts. Health conditions can also show more immediately in your nail bed. Doctors can usually detect a potentially serious condition just by looking at a person's nail bed. Some conditions, usually infections or traumas, will usually affect only one or two nails but systemic conditions will affect all of the nails. Doctors can sometimes tell if a person has heart, kidney, lung, connective tissue or liver diseases, diabetes, lupus just by looking at the fingernails and the nail beds. If you have any sudden changes or discolorations in your nails or your nail beds, please see a physician immediately as this can be symptomatic of something complex. Some conditions could be as simple as a vitamin or mineral deficiency, but it is always a good idea to have a doctor look at any changes that may not seem normal.

LIFESTYLE

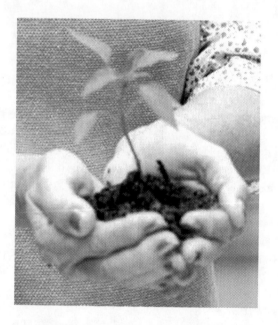

What is your lifestyle like? What you do with your hands plays a very important role in how long you can wear your nails. Here are some questions:

✓ Do you lift a lot of heavy objects?
✓ Do you type a lot?
✓ Do you garden? Without gloves?
✓ Are you the proverbial bull in the china shop, not watching where you place your hands, moving too fast and hitting objects with the tips of your fingers?

If you answered yes to these questions, you may want to keep your nails a little shorter or adjust your activity to compensate. You may have also noticed that there is a certain nail that always breaks. You may need to pay special attention to that nail. In most cases, there is usually something that you do with that nail that makes it susceptible to breaking.

A common complaint I would hear a lot about nails is "My nails peel!" There are reasons why nails peel.

- ✓ Are you in a lot of water and/or harsh chemicals without wearing rubber gloves?
- ✓ Do you use a nail clipper on dry nails?
- ✓ Do you pick at your nails or at your polish when it starts to chip?
- ✓ Have you had acrylic nails, gel nails or silk /fiberglass wraps? (Don't be fooled, they all cause damage to the natural nail!)
- ✓ How do you file your nails? Do you file from the edges to the tip or do you file back and forth? Do you file the tops of your nail when filing the edge?
- ✓ Do you drink enough water?
- ✓ Do you apply oil to your nails?

Bad habits and nervous habits play havoc with your nails. If you have thin nails that peel, and you work with harsh chemicals and lift a lot of heavy things, you can't expect your nails to be one inch long. Also consider that some conditions, such as thyroid problems, or medications, especially chemotherapy, have side effects that reflect in your nails.

The Nitty-Gritty

Now it's time to get down to business. There are a few rules when filing and shaping your nails. Remember what you learned about the nail structure, you'll need to remember that the nail is made of layers of flattened cells stacked one on top of another and held together with a cement like protein called keratin. It is when this cement is broken down at the tip of the nail that we get peeling. So how do we prevent this protein from being broken down? We use care in filing and shaping, we apply oil to keep the keratin flexible and we apply polish to hold the cells together that are vulnerable to peeling and wear.

Filing & Shaping

Some people can handle clipping their nails without any repercussions. These people have very moisturized and/or thin nails. For those that have nails that peel or split, do not use a nail clipper unless you have soaked your nails for a minimum of 2 minutes in warm water. When you clip your nails dry, you damage the "cement" thereby creating small cracks or gaps between the cells. Water softens the cement, so when you clip the nail it doesn't shatter the cement between the cells.

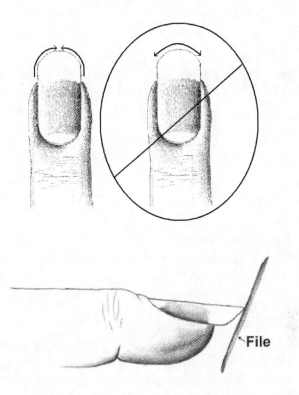

Always file your nails from the sides to the tip. Never file back and forth across the tip unless you are filing down a lot of length and only then you should finish up with filing from the sides to the tip. Hold your file, and file your nails at an angle, as shown above. This angle will aid in preventing peeling because you will be filing the layers from underneath the nail. You will also notice that there are fine "fringes" (like a frayed cloth) that hang from the underneath your nail and on top. Remove these "fringes" by gently filing or buffing them off. Always finish filing your nails with a very fine file, the finer the file, the better. This type of filing definitely will prevent peeling because you will be removing any pieces that can contribute to it.

Do not let the free edge of your nail grow much longer than one half of the nail bed length. The longer your free edge is, the more it puts stress on your nail. If your nails tend to break at a certain length, keep your nails just a little bit shorter than that. This way all of your nails can be the same length and look well manicured. Of course, there will be times that you will break a nail very low, just bear with it as it grows out. You can file some of the other nails down so the broken nail doesn't look as short.

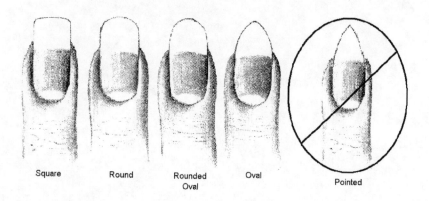

Square   Round   Rounded   Oval   Pointed
                    Oval

How you shape your nails is very individualistic, but I must point out that if you file your nails too pointed you increase your potential for breaking your nails because you reduce the stress area at the sides. Do not file your nails deep into the sides where the nail meets the flesh of the nail bed. The only time the sides of the nail should be filed narrowly is if the nail is extremely wide and only if you do not file the skin and damage the nail bed. If you have an oval to rounded cuticle area, you can file your nails as shown above. You can also try filing the tip of the nail to match what your cuticle area looks like, kind of like filing a mirror image. Sometimes this look can be very attractive, but keep in mind that all of your fingers are not going to be shaped the same around your cuticle. Pick the shape that appeals best and use that. You be the judge.

Nail Shapes That Mirror the Cuticle

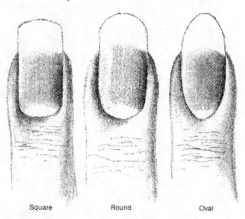

Square   Round   Oval

If you do get a break in your nail, don't be afraid to use nail glue. If there is peeling, it needs to be gently buffed off. This can be a little difficult because you don't want to buff any part of the natural nail that is healthy. Only buff the peeling portion smooth. If you buff too much, you'll wear down and thin the healthy part of the nail. The peeling nail has to eventually be filed completely off, that is the ONLY way to correct peeling nails. It is only then that your nails can be healthier. In time, we will be sealing in the tips of the peeling nails with polish. If your nails peel excessively, a nail strengthener may be necessary.

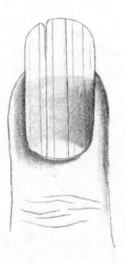

A little note on buffing the nails . . . If you have thin nails or nails with deep ridges, it is not suggested that you buff your nails. Buffing will only make thin nails thinner. If you have deep ridges, buffing will weaken your nails where the ridges were and then you may have the nail split down the center. Thin nails with ridges can be managed with a ridge filler base coat. If your nails are thick, you may find some benefits to buffing your nails because it will gently thin them out.

Moisture

As I mentioned earlier, your nails contain moisture, i.e. oil and water. The water content that is in the cells comes from your body and the water you drink. Eventually, some of this moisture will evaporate and the cells will become flatter and flatter. When you add layers of cuticle oil to the nail, it penetrates into the cement like protein and help to prevent some of this moisture in the cells from evaporating. This will aid to keep the nail flexible and keep the protein flexible. We need to topically apply the oil especially as we get older because we do not produce as much oil as we did when we were younger. Also, if you live in a dry climate, the moisture in your nails and cuticles will evaporate quicker than if you live in a humid environment. Lack of moisture in the nail is also one of the causes of vertical nail ridges and peeling. Remember what causes peeling? It is when this cement is broken down at the tip of the nail that we get peeling.

Oiling our nails with high-quality cuticle oil helps prevent this problem. For those saying, "I use a cuticle cream", or "I use a lotion every day", this will normally not penetrate through your polish let alone penetrate into your nail. Your body naturally doesn't secrete lotion, it secretes oil. Depending on the person and how dry their nails are is how often you need to apply cuticle oil. I usually suggest that oil be applied at least once a day and if the person has excessive peeling and ridges, 2-3 times per day. The hard part is getting into the habit. At night before bed is a good time to apply your cuticle oil. You don't need much oil, in fact, most people get their nails dripping in oil and that much is not necessary. If you apply a small amount and rub it in and go to the next nail and the next until the oil is barely visible.

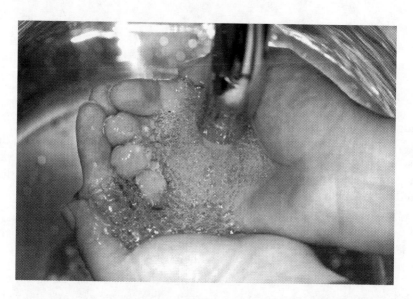

A second benefit we get from oiling our nails is that our nails do not absorb water as easily. When you have your hands in water for any period of time, what happens? Your skin prunes up. This is proof that your skin absorbs some of the water you're in. Your nails are made up of the same kind of cells that your skin is made of. So guess what happens to your nails when they have been in water for any period of time? They swell up! Water exposure is one of the causes of polish chipping and excessive water exposure is one of the causes of nails peeling. All of the expanding and contracting of the cement like protein, especially with hot water, creates small cracks, thereby creating peeling nails. So how do we repel the water and any potentially nasty chemicals that are in it away from your nails? We apply a high-quality cuticle oil so it can penetrate deeply into the nail. What happens when you combine oil and water? They don't mix. Now this doesn't mean that your nail will not absorb water, it just won't absorb as much.

A third benefit we get from oiling our nails is that our cuticles stay supple. This is an immediate benefit we get from oiling our nails. The other benefits take time to see the effects. If you oil your nails once a day, every day, you'll see some effects after a month, you'll really notice a difference after three months. The full effect usually takes about six months. That is how long it takes for the cells at your cuticle area to reach out to the tip of your nail. I did say that what I'm going to teach you was not a quick fix but you will still reap some of the benefits within a month's time.

Cuticles

Cuticles should be pushed back on a regular basis. It is best to push them back when they have been wet for a time. This softens the skin and makes it easier to push them back. Doing this after bathing or showering is a perfect time. Apply a cuticle remover to additionally soften the cuticle. Use a Cuticle pusher, cuticle stone or an Orangewood stick.

There are parts to the "cuticle" that you should know, especially when it comes to cutting it off. The skin around the nail, the Eponychium, Side Walls and Hyponychium, are seals that protect the nail from infection. Most people believe that their Eponychium is their cuticle, it isn't. Cuticle is the thin film of skin that sticks to your nail. When you push this cuticle back using a cuticle remover and cuticle pusher, it is usually not uniform in appearance. Sometimes, a good cuticle remover along with a cuticle stone can practically remove all of this dead skin, leaving a smooth seal around the Eponychium and the Side Walls. But do not overuse the stone on the nail surface as it will wear it down. Also, I have heard some people say that they have a nail growing under their fingernail, this is usually their Hyponychium. I've heard some people refer to it as their "quick". When the Hyponychium becomes hardened through lack of moisture, it can separate from the nail and increase the chance for infection to get under the nail.

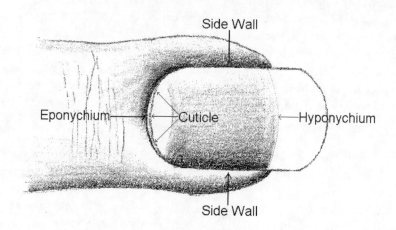

When it comes to cutting cuticles, you should only remove what is sticking out (i.e. hangnail or the thin film that was stuck to your nail). A hangnail is any skin that protrudes out and can tear deeper into the skin, creating an open wound. Also, some people get hangnails on the sides of their nails near the Side Walls. This type of hangnail can be trimmed off with cuticle nippers or gently filed off when your hands are dry. The trick to filing it off is to do it without filing the natural nail.

Polish

Normally, when you polish your nails, the polish will start to peel in approximately 2-3 days. How would you like to get 7-10 days wear from your polish? It's possible and I've even known women that have gotten *three* weeks wear from their polish with **NO CHIPPING & NO PEELING**!!! While I feel that three weeks is too much growth, the possibility of getting 2 weeks wear is highly appealing. In order to do this, there are a few things that need to be done to *prep* the nails and then to *maintain* them.

When it comes to polishing your nails, a woman should have a minimum of 2 coats of clear polish on her nails at all times to protect them from the elements and to add strength and thickness to the nail. If you wish to wear a color polish, use a base coat and a top coat with a minimum of 2 coats of colored polish. Be aware that 4 coats of polish will usually take an average of one hour to dry in order to not smudge them. If you have a hand for it, a French manicure is quite lovely, again using a base coat and a top coat. If you don't have a hand for a French manicure, try getting a white tip the old fashioned way, use a white pencil under the nail and then use a clear or sheer polish over your whole nail. The whole idea around wearing polish is that it protects your nail from external damage.

But before you can polish the nail, you must first prep it. Prepping means that you make certain there is no oil in between your natural nail and your base coat of polish. Have you ever seen polish peel up in one big sheet? That is because there was oil between the base coat and the natural nail. I know I said that it is important to oil your nails but oil doesn't belong on the surface of the nail just before the polish is applied. The oil can be removed with an oil-free polish remover, alcohol or just washing your hands well with soap and water. I personally prefer using a lint free wipe and acetone polish remover and/or alcohol. Besides removing oil from the main part of the nail, you also need to remove the oil from around the cuticle area and also from around the tip of the nail. Be certain to not touch your nails just before the polish is applied or you will put the oil back on your nails.

Also, not all nails need a nail strengthener and not all strengtheners are created equal. There are specific strengtheners for specific types of nails. There are nail strengtheners that work on thin nails that tear and/or peel. There are strengtheners for average nails hat have mild peeling. These are usually good for acrylic nail recovery. Some "strengtheners" help seal in moisture for dry, brittle nails. If your thick nails are peeling, sometimes a little cuticle oil will help along with keeping your polish on and "capped" at all times. For thicker nails or other nails that do not have any peeling, DO NOT use a nail strengthener. It's just not necessary. A simple natural nail base coat will do. There are even strengtheners for people with excessive peeling. For those people who have excessive peeling and have exhausted the other routes, there are strengtheners that go that extra step. It is a good idea to keep in mind that you should not be excessive with nail strengtheners. Strengtheners are not the only thing that makes a healthy nail strong, remember they need to be flexible as well.

When you apply polish, be careful not to get it into the cuticle. A heavy amount of polish in the cuticle also increases the risk of your polish peeling, but this time from the base of the nail. Polish does not have to be right next to, almost on the skin, to perform favorably or look good. Don't be afraid to have a thin line next to your cuticle that doesn't have any polish on it. The best way to keep polish out of your cuticle to begin with is to place your polish brush in the middle of your nail and then gently push it back towards the cuticle, keeping it just a hairline away from it. It is okay to have a good bit of polish on the brush but the trick is to keep it out of the cuticle. If you do happen to get the polish on your skin, have an orangewood stick available to remove it before it dries. Another trick to keep polish out of the cuticle is to apply your clear topcoat over the color polish you got on your skin and then wipe both off with an orangewood stick. If these tips still don't seem to help, a polish corrector pen will do the trick nicely.

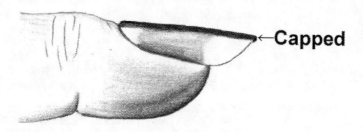

Also, when you polish your nails, it is important to "cap" your nails. This means that you will apply your polish in your normal fashion (from your cuticle area to your tip) and also apply your polish around the very tip of your nail where you file your nails. This will seal in the natural nail to protect it from wearing down and prevent the nail from peeling. Remember what was said earlier about water and how your nails swell when you have been in water for a time. Capping your nails will reduce how the nail swells.

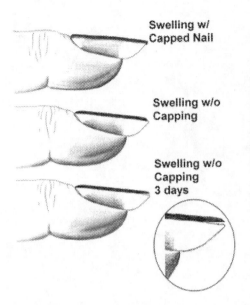

Swelling w/
Capped Nail

Swelling w/o
Capping

Swelling w/o
Capping
3 days

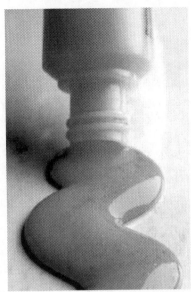

Here is the most important part to keep your polish on for longer than 2-3 days. You will need to maintain this "cap" by replacing it about every other day. The cap needs to be replaced because you wear it away as you touch things. Keep in mind that everything you touch acts as a natural nail file. Your clothing, the table top, the computer keyboard, and the worst one of all, paper! Replace the "cap" by applying more clear polish down your nails over your existing polish and around the very tip of the nail. Start this the day after you originally polished them. This will not only replace the cap, it will also add strength to your nail. It is this cap that will help keep your nail polish on longer.

One more thing about polish . . . Polish will smudge up to 15 minutes after application. Polish will also dent up to one hour and it takes a full twenty-four hours to *fully* set. It is important not to have your polished nails in water for prolonged periods of time or your polish will dry in the expanded state. This will make your polish peel in a sheet about the size of the free edge of your nail.

When you properly prep your nails, polish them with the techniques listed below, keeping them out of water for the first 24 hours, and by "capping" your nails with a clear coat of polish every other day, you will get 7-10 days wear from your polish. Don't believe me? Try it with red polish or the darkest color you like to wear. You'll love the results!

How to Polish

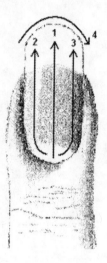

When polishing the nail, it works best to use the three stroke method down the nail on top of the nail. Here, however, we will add a forth stroke, around the tip of the nail. This forth stroke will be done for the base coat of polish, the first coat of color and the top coat.

Four Stroke Method

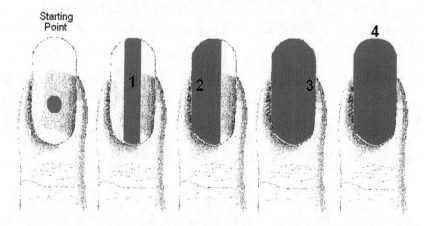

Also, to help keep the polish out of the cuticle, you will have a starting point on the nail. The whole idea of the starting point is if you have too much polish on the brush, you will be able to manage it better. The idea of applying polish correctly is to keep the polish out of the cuticle. The starting point helps to prevent this. Also the angle that you hold your brush is important in how the product is displaced. If you want your polish away from your cuticle, it takes practice and control. The control is used in resting your hand, pinkie and/or ring finger on something solid while polishing.

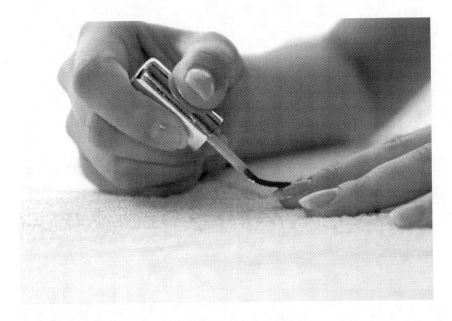

Follow the simple steps for polishing the nails, remembering to rest your hand on something, and with a little practice, you can even polish your nails quite well with your opposite hand.

How to Stroke on Polish

Try to use smooth movements

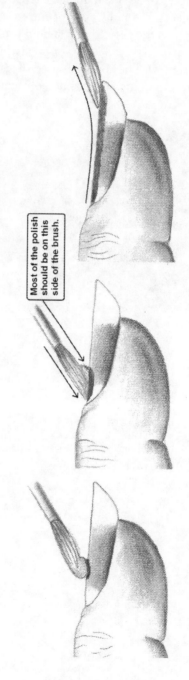

Most of the polish should be on this side of the brush.

With a small pool of polish at the tip of the brush, slowly push the brush toward the cuticle, flattening and fanning the brush til it makes a straight edge at the base of the nail.

After fanning out the brush, the polish should be a hair-line away from the cuticle. If the polish should get on the cuticle or skin, remove it with an orangewood stick.

Slowly pull the polish out toward the tip of the nail.

Natural Nail Repair

If you crack your nail, don't be afraid to use nail glue. If the crack is very bad, use a little filler powder with your nail glue and smooth it down as best as you can with a fine file. The idea is to build up the area where the crack is and file it flush with the natural nail. If the nail breaks again in the same spot, you can just re-glue it. To remove the glue and filler once the crack has grown out or if it needs to be replaced, soak it in acetone. Remember that glue and acetone dry out the nail. A second repair option is a product called Crack Attacker ™. This is a clear adhesive backed band aid that goes over polish. Place the Crack Attacker ™ at the edge of the nail where the break is, covering the break. I recommend that you do not use the Crack Attacker ™ on a bare nail. This is because, when you remove it, you could remove a few layers of nail plate with the bandage.

Another old fashioned, but effective, way to repair the nail without any damage is to use a "paper patch". A paper patch is a thin paper, usually a clean teabag, eyeglass paper or thin coffee filter, used in conjunction with a ridge filler base coat. Apply your ridge filler or base coat to a clean nail. Press a small, clean paper over the crack, leaving a very small amount that can be tucked around the edge of the nail to seal in the crack. Make sure that there are no bubbles and that the edges are tacked down. Let this first coat dry then apply 1 to 2 coats of ridge filler over the paper, making certain that the paper's edges stay down. It is usually a good idea to tear the paper before applying it instead of cutting it. A torn edge will help the paper blend better than a straight edge. You can also lightly buff the patch with the polish on it to smooth down any rough edges before you apply your color polish. A paper patch needs to be replaced if re-broken or if you change your polish.

PEDICURES

Toenails are no different than fingernails except that you are usually not trying to grow any length and, for most people, it is difficult to do a pedicure on yourself. Polishing the feet takes good eye sight, flexibility and a lot of patience. For this reason, it is usually best to have a pedicure professionally done or to have a friend do your toes. If you should decide to do it yourself, keep the following in mind.

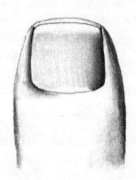

Cutting and filing your toenails is no different than your fingernails, except toenails are usually thicker and harder to cut. This is when it is crucial that you soak your toenails for a *minimum* of two minutes before cutting them. Be careful not to cut your toenails too short! It is best if you do not cut your toenail below the nail fold. Most people cut their nails too short. Cutting your nails too short can lead to many problems, such as ingrown toenails and infections. Remember, just because there is white at the tip of your toe does not mean that you cut it off. Also, if a toenail is thicker, sometimes you can file it thinner. Use care that you do not mistake a strong c-curve on your toenail for a thick toenail. It can be very painful if you thin out the wrong nail.

Cleaning the cuticle is done the same way as on the fingers. Sometimes the cuticle and the Eponychium grow heavier on the toes, especially the pinkie toe. Trim it off if it is too large, but be careful you do not break the skin by cutting too deeply.

Callus files are really important in the care of the foot. Some callus files work better on dry feet than on wet feet. There are even Microplanes for the feet if you have thick hard callus. These are just like the cheese graters and wood shavers that are out on the market but these are made just for callus. Again, use care with these as you can really hurt yourself if you go down too far. If you use a very coarse callus file, be sure to smooth it out with a finer callus file as to prevent the skin from snagging on clothing, sheets, carpeting, etc. The skin should be smooth to the touch.

To properly moisturize the feet, it is best to use heavier creams that are made specifically for them. Creams that contain urea do the best job in moisturizing the feet, especially dry cracked feet. Depending on how dry your feet get, you should moisturize callus often. Some people need to moisturize at least once, or even twice a day. Most lotions that are made for the hands and body don't do much to moisturize the feet properly.

If you have athletes foot, there are topical creams and sprays that you can buy over the counter. There is even a fungus that mimics dry feet. If you have tried all kinds of creams and lotions with no success, try an antifungal treatment in conjunction with your moisturizing lotion. Things like planters' warts, fungus toenails and unknown foot conditions need care from a physician. Be aware that over the counter products for a true toenail fungus usually only have a 1-2% cure rate. It is better to go to the physician/podiatrist and get a prescription. The prescriptions have up to a 68% cure rate for fungus toenails, but the doctor may need to monitor your liver for internal medications.

Summary

I would like to thank you for reading this publication and hope you find it very useful. Some of the information here can seem confusing but I think I made this as easy to understand as possible. All it takes is to create good nail habits. Remember, it takes three weeks to create a good habit and only 3 days to break it. If you follow the information I've presented here, you should never have to wear artificial nails again. Your nails should recover from peeling provided there is not an internal catalyst. There are occasions when you try to very hard and use all the right products, you still can't get rid of peeling nails, nothing seems to work. This is when you need to realize that some conditions, such as thyroid problems, or medications, especially chemotherapy, have side effects. It is best to talk with your physician if you continue to have problems.

There really is no substitute for a good professional manicure or pedicure, they are a real pleasure, and at times, very necessary. A professional nail tech can usually do a better job of cutting cuticle and polishing the nail than you can. They can also give you added advice on your nails and your nail care. If you should decide on getting a professional manicure and/or pedicure in between your own at home care, please be aware that not all nail techs or nail salons are created equal. Ask friends, neighbors or co-workers for a referral of a nail tech or nail salon they would recommend. Quality nail technicians with conscientious sanitation standards are out there. With whomever you decide to go to, if you are uncertain about their sanitation procedures, feel free to bring your own implements. If you do keep your own implements, it is also a good idea to keep them clean yourself. Wash them and wipe them down with alcohol. This way you can be sure that your own implements are clean. Feel free to discuss their sanitation procedures and always check for their license. If you feel there is an issue with the cleanliness of the salon, or feel that they have broken a law of some kind, please contact the Board of Cosmetology for that state to lodge a complaint. The phone number, addresses and some of the websites for the different governing boards are listed at the end of this book for your convenience. If enough consumers are aware and educated about what to watch out for, cleanliness issues and personal discomfort should become things of the past.

Please feel free to visit my website at www.bella10.com. I hope to continue to have more information about nail care and the nail service industry for you.

Bonus Facts

Here are some interesting facts about natural nails:

✓ The free edge of the nail will reflect a person's general health at the time it was initially created in the nail matrix.

✓ A pregnant woman's nails will grow faster than a woman who is not pregnant.

✓ Nails grow faster in the summer than in the winter.

✓ Nails (and hands) usually dry out, crack and/or peel in the winter.

✓ Nails grow slower as we get older.

✓ The longer the finger, the faster the nail grows.

✓ Buffing will thin the natural nail.

✓ Small white spots on the nail are usually caused by the nail being bumped or other minor injury (i.e. caught in a drawer).

✓ Natural nails will develop hang nails on the sides of the fingers faster than someone with artificial nails.

Here are some interesting facts about polish:

✓ Polish can protect the nails from the elements and from usage.

✓ You damage and thin your nails every time you peel your polish off your natural nails. Doing this removes a layer of nail plate.

✓ Some color polishes will stain the natural nail; this can be gently buffed out if necessary.

✓ Base coat adheres better to the natural nail better because it is more flexible than color polish or top coat.

✓ Some people are allergic to Formaldehyde in polish, but this is usually rare.

✓ Formaldehyde in polish hardens and adds shine to the polish.

- ✓ Too much formaldehyde in a polish can dry out the nails, especially if the person is sensitive to formaldehyde to begin with.
- ✓ Polish that contains Formaldehyde and Toluene will not chip as fast as polishes that do not. However, there are constantly new formulations in Formaldehyde/Toluene/BDP free polishes that may prove to have just as much wearability.
- ✓ It is always better to purchase professional brand polishes than over the counter polishes. Remember, you get what you pay for.

Here are some interesting facts about artificial nails:

- ✓ Any kind of artificial nail (acrylic, gel, silk or fiberglass wraps) will damage the nail.
- ✓ Improper drilling of artificial nails will cause "rings of fire". This is where the nail has been thinned almost down through the nail to the nail bed itself.
- ✓ Improper care of artificial nails will usually cause a bacterial infection.
- ✓ What most people think is a fungus on their fingernails is usually a bacterial infection.
- ✓ Artificial nails can be applied with a minimal damage if the nail tech makes the effort not to damage the nail.
- ✓ To remove Acrylic nails and glue/resin based products, they should *always* be soaked off with a nail remover or acetone.
- ✓ If an artificial nail is picked, pried, or ripped off it increases the damage to the natural nail.
- ✓ Acetone will dry out the nails, if you use it to remove artificial nails be sure to use oil immediately afterward.
- ✓ When artificial nails are removed the natural nails are usually soft and will harden up within a 24 hour time period.
- ✓ Acrylic fumes/vapors are not dangerous, they just smell bad.
- ✓ Technicians use masks when doing acrylic nails because of the dust, not the vapors.

Here are some interesting facts about licensing and sanitation in nail salons:

- ✓ Most states require a minimum of a nail technician/manicurist license to perform nail services
- ✓ Cosmetologist license is also valid to perform nail services

✓ Connecticut is the only state that does not require a license to perform manicuring services. However, a cosmetologist license is required to perform pedicures.

✓ In Canada, a nail technician license is required in the following provinces; British Columbia, Manitoba, New Brunswick and Nova Scotia.

✓ In U.S. Territories, Guam requires a manicurist license and Puerto Rico requires a cosmetologist license.

✓ As of 2007, it is expressly prohibited for a Nail Technician/Manicurist to cut skin (i.e. callus, corns) especially with the use of a razor or Credo blade in the following states:

- o Arizona
- o California
- o Connecticut
- o District of Columbia
- o Florida
- o Kentucky
- o Maryland
- o Massachusetts
- o Michigan
- o Mississippi
- o Montana
- o Nebraska
- o New Hampshire
- o New Jersey
- o New Mexico
- o New York
- o North Carolina
- o Pennsylvania
- o Rhode Island
- o South Dakota
- o Wisconsin

✓ Most states (except Connecticut) require some kind of immersion sanitation procedure for implements. Most require a hospital grade disinfectant, or EPA-registered disinfectant. Some states also allow the use of bleach solutions and 70% alcohol. For a complete list of sanitation requirements go to www.bella10.com

✓ Sanitation solutions are best when they are bactericidal, virucidal, fungicidal, tuberculocidal, and effective against HIV and Hepatitis C

✓ If an implement cannot be sanitized, it should be disposable.

✓ Sanitized implements should usually be kept in a dry container or drawer, free from contaminants.

✓ Pedicure spa chairs should be cleaned and sanitized with a hospital grade disinfectant for 10 minutes and then rinsed with clean water between each client.

✓ Each state has its own state board and laws governing manicurists/nail technicians and the salons they work in.

✓ If you have a complaint about a nail salon or a nail technician that you believe has violated a state law or a state mandated sanitation practice, you have the right to contact their state's governing agency.

Procedures

Manicure

1. Remove old polish from both hands
2. Shape your nails on both hands in the desired shape

   a. Be sure to even the length of all your nails

3. Place hand in warm soapy water to soften and clean the cuticle
4. After two minutes, remove your hand from the finger bowl and apply cuticle remover
5. Push back cuticle, clean under the nail and nip off any loose cuticle or hangnails
6. Repeat steps 3 through 6 on your second hand
7. Use a good scrub on your hands and rinse off
8. Apply hand lotion to both hands
9. Clean nail plate on both hands to remove any surface oils and apply polish

   a. Base coat
   b. Color polish
   c. Top coat

10. After 1 minute, apply nail dryer

11. After 10-15 minutes, treat cuticles with cuticle oil

Pedicure

1. Remove old polish from both feet
2. Use a callus file on the bottom of both feet

   a. If your callus is heavy

      i. Use a Microplane
      ii. Or coarse callus file
      iii. Be certain to finish with a fine callus file

   b. If your callus is minimal

      i. Use a medium/fine callus file

3. Soak your feet in warm soapy water
4. Cut and file your nails on your first foot to the desired shape

   a. Be sure not to cut the nails too short

5. Apply cuticle remover
6. Push back cuticle, clean under the nail and nip off any loose cuticle or hangnails
7. Repeat steps 4 through 6 on your second foot
8. Apply an scrub to both feet and rinse off
9. Apply a good foot cream
10. Clean nail plate on both feet to remove any surface oil and apply polish

    a. Base coat
    b. Color polish
    c. Top coat

11. After 1 minute, apply nail dryer
12. After 10-15 minutes, treat cuticles with cuticle oil

LIST OF GOVERNING AGENCIES

United States

ALABAMA

Alabama Board of Cosmetology
Address: PO Box 301750, Montgomery, AL 36130
Phone: (334) 242-1918; (800) 815-7453
Web: www.aboc.state.al.us

ALASKA

Alaska Barbers & Hairdressers
Address: PO Box 110806, Juneau, AK 99811-0806
Phone: (907) 465-2547
Web: www.commerce.state.ak.us /occ/pbah.htm

ARIZONA

Arizona Board of Cosmetology
Address: 1721 E. Broadway, Tempe, AZ 85282
Phone: (480) 784-4539 ext. 227
Web: www.azboc.gov

ARKANSAS

Arkansas State Board of Cosmetology
Address: 101 E. Capitol Ave. #108, Little Rock, AR 72201
Phone: (501) 682-2168
Web: www.arkansas.gov/cos

CALIFORNIA

California Dept. of Consumer Affairs Board of Barbering & Cosmetology
Address: PO Box 944226, Sacramento, CA 94244-2260
Phone: (916) 445-0916; (800) 952-5210 (CA only)
Web: www.barbercosmo.ca.gov

COLORADO
Colorado Barbers & Cosmetology Licensure
Address: 1560 Broadway #1350, Denver, CO 80202
Phone: (303) 894-7772
Web: www.dora.state.co.us/barbers_cosmetologists

CONNECTICUT
Connecticut Dept. of Public Health
Address: 410 Capitol Ave., MS # 13 PHO PO Box 340308, Hartford, CT 06134-0308
Phone: (860) 509-7648
Web: www.ct.gov/dph/cwp/view.asp?a=3143&q=388878

DELAWARE
Delaware State Board of Cosmetology & Barbering
Address: 861 Silver Lake Blvd. #203, Dover, DE 19904
Phone: (302)744-4500
Web: www.dpr.delaware.gov/boards/cosmetology/index.shtml

DISTRICT OF COLUMBIA
District of Columbia Cosmetology & Barbering
Address: 941 N. Capital St. Room 7200, Washington, DC 20002
Phone: (202) 442-4400
Web: www.asisvcs.com/indhome_fs.asp?CPCAT=2009STATEREG

FLORIDA
Florida Board of Cosmetology
Address: 1940 N. Monroe St., Tallahassee, FL 32399-0790
Phone: (850) 487-1395
Web: www.myflorida.com/dbpr/pro/cosmo/documents/cosmo_faq.pdf

GEORGIA
Georgia State Board of Cosmetology
Address: 237 Coliseum Drive, Macon, GA 31208-3858
Phone: (478) 207-2440
Web: sos.georgia.gov/plb/cosmetology/default.htm

HAWAII
Hawaii Board of Barbering & Cosmetology
Address: PO Box 3469, Honolulu, HI 96801
Phone: (808) 587-3295
Web: hawaii.gov/dcca/areas/pvl/boards/barber/

IDAHO
Idaho State Board of Cosmetology
Address: 1109 Main St. #220, Boise, ID 83702
Phone: (208) 334-3233
Web: ibol.idaho.gov/cos.htm

ILLINOIS

Illinois Dept. of Professional Regulation

Address: 320 W. Washington St., 3rd Floor, Springfield, IL 62786
Phone: (217) 785-0800
Web: www.idfpr.com/dpr/WHO/nailtec.asp

INDIANA

Indiana State Board of Cosmetology Examiners

Address: 402 W. Washington, Room W072, Indianapolis, IN 46204
Phone: (317) 234-3031
Web: www.in.gov/pla/cosmo.htm

IOWA

Iowa Cosmetology Board of Examiners—Dept. of Public Health/ Professional Licensure

Address: 321 E. 12th St. Lucas Bldg., 5th Floor, Des Moines, IA 50319-0075
Phone: (515) 281-4416
Web: www.idph.state.ia.us/licensure/board_home.asp?board=cos

KANSAS

Kansas Board of Cosmetology

Address: 714 SW Jackson St. #100, Topeka, KS 66603
Phone: (785) 296-3155
Web: www.kansas.gov/kboc

KENTUCKY

Kentucky State Board of Hairdressers & Cosmetologists

Address: 111 St. James Ct. #A, Frankfort, KY 40601
Phone: (502) 564-4262
Web: www.kbhc.ky.gov/

LOUISIANA

Louisiana State Board of Cosmetology

Address: 11622 Sunbelt Ct., Baton Rouge, LA 70809
Phone: (225) 756-3404
Web: www.lsbc.louisiana.gov/

MAINE

Maine Board of Barbering & Cosmetology

Address: 35 State House Station, Augusta, ME 04333
Phone: (207) 624-8603
Web: www.maine.gov/pfr/professionallicensing/professions/barbers/index.htm

MARYLAND

Maryland Board of Cosmetologists

Address: 500 N. Calvert St., Room 201, Baltimore, MD 21202
Phone: (410) 230-6320
Web: www.dllr.state.md.us/license/occprof/cos.html

MASSACHUSETTS
Massachusetts Board of Cosmetology
Address: 239 Causaway St., #500, Boston, MA 02114
Phone: (617) 727-9940
Web: www.state.ma.us/reg/boards/hd

MICHIGAN
Michigan Dept. of Consumer & Industry Svcs., Board of Cosmetology
Address: PO Box 30018, Lansing, MI 48909
Phone: (517) 241-9288
Web: www.michigan.gov/dleg/0,1607,7-154-35299_35414_35459—,00.html

MINNESOTA
Minnesota Barber & Cosmetologist Examiners Board
Address: 2829 University Ave. SE #710, Minneapolis, MN 55414
Phone: (651) 201-2742
Web: www.bceboard.state.mn.us

MISSISSIPPI
Mississippi State Board of Cosmetology
Address: PO Box 55689, Jackson, MS 39296-5689
Phone: (601) 354-5315
Web: www.msbc.state.ms.us

MISSOURI
Missouri State Board of Cosmetology
Address: PO Box 1062, Jefferson City, MO 65102
Phone: (573) 751-1052
Web: www.pr.mo.gov/cosbar.asp

MONTANA
Montana Board of Cosmetologists
Address: PO Box 200513, Helena, MT 59620-0513
Phone: (406) 841-2335
Web: www.discoveringmontana.com/dli/cos

NEBRASKA
Nebraska State Board of Cosmetology Examiners/Credentialing Division
Address: PO Box 95026, Lincoln, NE 68509-5026
Phone: (402) 471-2117
Web: www.hhs.state.ne.us/CRL/mhcs/cosindex.htm

NEVADA
Nevada State Board of Cosmetology
Address: 1785 E. Sahara Ave. #255, Las Vegas, NV 89104
Phone: (702) 486-6542
Web: www.cosmetology.nv.gov

NEW HAMPSHIRE
New Hampshire Board of Barbering, Cosmetology & Esthetics
Address: 2 Industrial Park Dr., Concord, NH 03301
Phone: (603) 271-3608
Web: www.nh.gov/cosmet

NEW JERSEY
New Jersey Board of Cosmetology & Hairstyling
Address: PO Box 45003, Newark, NJ 07101
Phone: (973) 504-6400
Web: www.state.nj.us/oag/ca/nonmedical/coshair.htm

NEW MEXICO
New Mexico Board of Barbers & Cosmetologists
Address: 2550 Cerrillos Rd., PO Box 25101, Santa Fe, NM 87504
Phone: (505) 476-4690
Web: www.rld.state.nm.us/BarbersCosmetologists/index.html

NEW YORK
New York Dept. of State, Licensing Svcs. Division
Address: PO Box 22001, Albany, NY 12201-2001
Phone: (518) 474-4429
Web: www.dos.state.ny.us/lcns/professions/appearance/appear.htm

NORTH CAROLINA
North Carolina Board of Cosmetology
Address: 1201 Front St. #110, Raleigh, NC 27609
Phone: (919) 733-4117
Web: www.cosmetology.state.nc.us

NORTH DAKOTA
North Dakota State Board of Cosmetology
Address: PO Box 2177, Bismarck, ND 58502-2177
Phone: (701) 224-9800
Web: www.beautyschoolsdirectory.com/faq/license_nd.php

OHIO
Ohio State Board of Cosmetology
Address: 1929 Gateway Circle, Grove City, Ohio 43123
Phone: (614) 466-3834
Web: www.cos.ohio.gov

OKLAHOMA
Oklahoma Board of Cosmetology
Address: 2401 NW 23rd St. #84, Oklahoma City, OK 73107
Phone: (405) 521-2441
Web: www.cosmo.state.ok.us/

OREGON
Oregon Health Licensing Office Board of Cosmetology
Address: 700 Summer St. NE #320, Salem, OR 97301-1287
Phone: (503) 378-8667; (503) 373-2114 (TDD)
Web: www.oregon.gov/OHLA/COS/index.shtml

PENNSYLVANIA
Pennsylvania State Board of Cosmetology
Address: PO Box 2649, Harrisburg, PA 17105-2649
Phone: (717) 783-7130
Web: www.dos.state.pa.us/bpoa/cwp/view.asp?a=1104&q=432561

RHODE ISLAND
Rhode Island Board of Hairdressing & Barbering
Address: 3 Capitol Hill, Room 104, Providence, RI 02908
Phone: (401) 222-2827
Web: www.health.ri.gov/hsr/professions/hair_barb.php

SOUTH CAROLINA
South Carolina Board of Cosmetology
Address: PO Box 11329, Columbia, SC 29211
Phone: (803) 896-4568
Web: www.llronline.com/POL/Cosmetology/

SOUTH DAKOTA
South Dakota Cosmetology Commission
Address: 500 E. Capitol, Pierre, SD 57501
Phone: (605) 773-6193
Web: www.state.sd.us/dol/boards/cos

TENNESSEE
Tennessee State Board of Cosmetology
Address: 500 James Robertson Pkwy., Room 130, Nashville, TN 37243-1147
Phone: (615) 741-2515
Web: tennessee.gov/commerce/boards/cosmo/

TEXAS
Texas Dept. of Licensing & Regulation
Address: PO Box 12157, Austin, TX 78711
Phone: (512) 463-6599; (800) 803-9202 (TX only)
Web: www.license.state.tx.us/cosmet/cosmet.htm

UTAH
Utah Board of Cosmetology
Address: 160 E. 300 South, PO Box 146741, Salt Lake City, UT 84114-6741
Phone: (801) 530-6628; (866) 275-3675 (in Utah)
Web: www.dopl.utah.gov/licensing/cosmetology_barbering.html

VERMONT

Vermont Board of Barbers & Cosmetology
Address: National Life Bldg North FL2, Montpelier, VT 05620-3402
Phone: (802) 828-1134
Web: www.vtprofessionals.org/opr1/cosmetologists/

VIRGINIA

Virginia Board for Barbers & Cosmetology
Address: 9960 Mayland Dr., #400, Richmond, VA 23233-1463
Phone: (804) 367-8509
Web: www.dpor.virginia.gov/dporweb/bnc_main.cfm

WASHINGTON

Washington Board of Cosmetologists, Barbers, Manicurists & Estheticians
Address: PO Box 9026, Olympia, WA 98507-9026
Phone: (360) 664-6626
Web: www.dol.wa.gov/business/cosmetology/index.html

WEST VIRGINIA

West Virginia Board of Barbers & Cosmetologists
Address: 1716 Pennsylvania Ave. #7, Charleston, WV 25302
Phone: (304) 558-2924
Web: www.wvdhhr.org/wvbc/

WISCONSIN

Wisconsin Barbering & Cosmetology Examining Board
Address: 1400 E. Washington Ave. PO Box 8935, Madison, WI 53708
Phone: (608) 266-5511
Web: drl.wi.gov/boards/bac/index.htm

WYOMING

Wyoming State Board of Cosmetology
Address: 2515 Warren Ave. #302, Cheyenne, WY 82002
Phone: (307) 777-3534
Web: cosmetology.state.wy.us/

U.S. Territories

GUAM
Guam Board of Barbering & Cosmetology
Address: PO Box 2816, Hagatna, GU 96932
Phone: (671) 735-7406
Web: (none)

PUERTO RICO
Puerto Rico Secretaría Auxiliar de Juntas Examindoras
Address: PO Box 9023271, San Juan, PR 00902-3271
Phone: (787) 722-2121
Web: www.estado.gobierno.pr

Canada

ALBERTA
Alberta Dept. of Advanced Education & Career Development/Beauty Consultant Division
Address: 10030 107th St., 7th Floor, Edmonton, AB T5J 4X7
Phone: (780) 427-8517
Web: www.tradesecrets.org

BRITISH COLUMBIA
British Columbia Board of Examiners, Cosmetologists Assn. of British Columbia
Address: 899 W. 8th Ave., Vancouver, BC V5Z 1E3
Phone: (604) 871-0222 ext. 303; (800) 663-9283
Web: www.cabccanada.com

MANITOBA
Manitoba Department of Education, Apprenticeship, Advanced Education & Training
Address: 1010 401 York Ave., Winnipeg, MB R3C 0P8
Phone: (204) 945-5436
Web: www.edu.gov.mb.ca/apprenticeship

NEW BRUNSWICK
New Brunswick Cosmetology Association
Address: 299 York St., Fredericton, NB E3B 3P2
Phone: (506) 458-8087
Web: www.canb.ca/

NEWFOUNDLAND
Newfoundland Industrial Training Division, Dept. of Youth Services & Post-Secondary Training
Address: PO Box 8700, St. John's, NF A1B 4J6
Phone: (709) 729-5636
Web: www.gov.nf.ca/edu/post/app.htm

NORTHWEST TERRITORIES
Northwest Territories Dept. of Education, Culture & Employment
Address: Career Centre, Box 1320, Yellowknife, NWT X1A 2L9
Phone: (867) 873-7357
Web: www.gov.nt.ca

NOVA SCOTIA
Cosmetology Assn. of Nova Scotia
Address: 126 Chain Lake Dr., Halifax, NS B3S 1A2
Phone: (902) 468-6477; (800) 765-8757
Web: www.nscosmetology.ca

ONTARIO
Ontario Ministry of Education, Training, Colleges & Universities
Address: 900 Bay St., Toronto, ON M7A 1L2
Phone: (416) 325-2929
Web: www.edu.gov.on.ca

SASKETCHEWAN
Sasketchewan Dept. of Education/Apprenticeship Division
Address: 2140 Hamilton St., Regina, SK S4P 3V7
Phone: (306) 787-2444
Web: www.saskapprenticeship.ca

YUKON
Yukon Government of Yukon, Corporate Affairs
Address: PO Box 2703, C-6, Whitehorse, YK Y1A 2C6
Phone: (867) 667-5314
Web: www.community.gov.yk.ca/corp/index.html